ICS 11.020

SCM

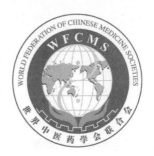

世界中医药学会联合会

World Federation of Chinese Medicine Societies

SCM 69–2021

国际中医技术操作规范
醒脑开窍针刺法治疗中风

International Standardized Manipulations of Chinese Medicine
Xingnao Kaiqiao Acupuncture for Stroke

U0297479

世界中联国际组织标准
International Standard of WFCMS

2021–12–16 发布实施
Issued & implemented on December.16, 2021

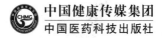
中国健康传媒集团
中国医药科技出版社

图书在版编目（CIP）数据

国际中医技术操作规范.醒脑开窍针刺法治疗中风 / 世界中医药学会联合会著.—北京：中国医药
科技出版社，2022.9

ISBN 978-7-5214-3364-7

Ⅰ.①国…　Ⅱ.①世…　Ⅲ.①中风 – 针刺疗法 – 技术操作规程 – 中国 – 汉、英　Ⅳ.① R21-65

中国版本图书馆 CIP 数据核字（2022）第 160758 号

美术编辑　陈君杞
版式设计　南博文化

出版　**中国健康传媒集团** | 中国医药科技出版社

地址　北京市海淀区文慧园北路甲 22 号

邮编　100082

电话　发行：010-62227427　邮购：010-62236938

网址　www.cmstp.com

规格　880×1230 mm $^1/_{16}$

印张　1 $^3/_4$

字数　46 千字

版次　2022 年 9 月第 1 版

印次　2022 年 9 月第 1 次印刷

印刷　北京紫瑞利印刷有限公司

经销　全国各地新华书店

书号　ISBN 978-7-5214-3364-7

定价　**29.00 元**

获取新书信息、投稿、
为图书纠错，请扫码
联系我们。

目　次

前言 ·· III

引言 ·· IV

1 范围 ··· 1

2 规范性引用文件 ··· 1

3 术语和定义 ··· 1

4 施术前准备 ··· 2

    4.1 针具选择 ··· 2

    4.2 体位选择 ··· 2

    4.3 腧穴定位 ··· 2

    4.4 消毒 ·· 2

    4.5 环境要求 ··· 2

5 主穴 ··· 2

    5.1 治疗原则 ··· 2

    5.2 应用范围 ··· 2

    5.3 主穴 I 操作 ·· 2

    5.4 主穴 II 操作 ··· 3

6 辅穴 ··· 3

    6.1 治疗原则 ··· 3

    6.2 应用范围 ··· 3

    6.3 辅穴 I 操作 ·· 3

    6.4 辅穴 II 操作 ··· 3

7 合并症治疗 ··· 4

    7.1 吞咽障碍 ··· 4

    7.2 语言障碍 ··· 4

    7.3 肩手综合征 ··· 4

    7.4 手指功能障碍 ·· 4

    7.5 足内翻 ··· 4

8 注意事项 ·· 5

9 禁忌 ··· 5

附录 A（资料性）醒脑开窍针刺法的含义 ·· 6

参考文献 ··· 7

Foreword ·· 8

Introduction ··· 9

1 Scope ··· 10

2 Normative references ·· 10

3 Terms and definitions ··· 10

4 Preparations before treatment ··· 11

4.1 Needle selection ··· 11

4.2 Posture selection ·· 11

4.3 Acupoint positioning ·· 12

4.4 Disinfection ·· 12

4.5 Treatment area requirements ·· 12

5 Primary acupoints ··· 12

5.1 Treatment principles ··· 12

5.2 Scope of application ·· 12

5.3 Technique for primary acupoints-Set Ⅰ ·· 12

5.4 Technique for primary acupoints-Set Ⅱ ·· 13

6 Auxiliary acupoints ·· 13

6.1 Treatment principles ··· 13

6.2 Scope of application ·· 13

6.3 Technique for auxiliary acupoints-Set Ⅰ ··· 13

6.4 Technique for auxiliary acupoints-Set Ⅱ ··· 13

7 Treatment for complications ·· 14

7.1 Dysphagia ··· 14

7.2 Aphasia ··· 14

7.3 Shoulder-hand syndrome ··· 14

7.4 Finger function impairment ·· 15

7.5 Strephenopodia ··· 15

8 Precautions ··· 16

9 Contraindications ··· 16

Annex A (Informative) Explanation of Xingnao Kaiqiao Acupuncture ····················· 17

References ··· 19

前　言

请注意本文件的某些内容可能涉及专利。本文件的发布机构不承担识别专利的责任。

主要起草单位：天津中医药大学第一附属医院、国家中医针灸临床医学研究中心。

参与起草单位（排名不分先后）：重庆市中医院、宁夏回族自治区中医医院暨中医研究院、深圳市宝安区中医院、美国亚利桑那州针灸研究所、英国梅德斯通中医中心、德国慕尼黑中医诊所、马来西亚国家癌症中心。

主要起草人：石学敏。

参与起草人及审阅专家（按姓氏拼音排序）：

中国：卞金玲、常颖慧、戴晓乔、杜宇征、郭扬、李礼、刘健、史慧妍、王璨、王竹行、肖凌勇、于澜、张超、赵琦。

美国：刘静。

英国：赵俊红。

德国：Florian von Damnitz。

马来西亚：钟尚烨。

本文件起草程序遵守了世界中医药学会联合会发布的《世界中联国际组织标准管理办法》和SCM 0001-2009《标准制定和发布工作规范》。

本文件由世界中医药学会联合会发布，版权归世界中医药学会联合会所有。

引　言

　　本文件制定的目的在于规范醒脑开窍针刺法的临床操作，指导相关医师正确使用本针法，以保障醒脑开窍针刺法规范应用于针灸临床、教育、科研等，确保其安全性、有效性，以便更好地推动醒脑开窍针刺法的国际推广与应用。

　　针灸能够产生良好临床疗效的关键在于针刺手法，刺激量是影响临床疗效的重要因素。历代医家都对针刺手法进行了朴素的定量分析，其中大多数基于主观经验，缺乏成熟和统一的客观定量标准。石学敏院士于1976年率先提出针刺手法量学概念，首次对针刺作用力方向、大小、施术时间、两次针刺间隔时间等针刺手法的四大要素进行了科学界定，使针刺手法更具规范性、可重复性与可操作性。

　　针刺操作过程中所涉及的刺激量参数，包括进针参数（方向、角度、深度等）、时间参数（介入时间、行针时间、留针时间、频次、疗程等）和行针参数（手法、幅度、频率等）。早期临床研究发现，规范手法量学组与非规范手法量学组相比，能够更好地改善中风患者的脑电图、脑血流、微循环、血液流变学等指标，促进患者运动功能、感觉功能、语言功能等恢复。近年功能影像研究提示：针刺手法是脑功能成像变化的关键影响因素。基础研究也证实：针刺行针时间和捻转频率是影响针刺疗效的重要因素，不同针刺手法参数具有各自特异性调控的生物学途径。

　　因此，科学的手法量学标准是保证针刺效应最大化的必要条件，而开展针刺手法量学研究是针刺规范化、标准化的必由之路。

国际中医技术操作规范　醒脑开窍针刺法治疗中风

1　范围

本文件规定了醒脑开窍针刺法治疗中风的术语和定义、治疗原则、应用范围、腧穴组方、操作步骤与要求、注意事项与禁忌等。

本文件适用于醒脑开窍针刺法治疗中风的临床技术操作。

2　规范性引用文件

下列文件中的内容通过文中的规范性引用而构成本文件必不可少的条款。凡是标注日期的引用文件，仅该日期对应的版本适用于本文件。凡是未标注日期的引用文件，其最新版本（包括所有的修改单）适用于本文件。

GB 2024-2016　针灸针

GB/T 12346-2021　经穴名称与定位

GB 15982-2012　医院卫生消毒标准

GB/T 16751.1-1997　中医临床诊疗术语第1部分：疾病

GB/T 21709.4-2008　针灸技术操作规范第4部分：三棱针

GB/T 21709.20-2009　针灸技术操作规范第20部分：毫针基本刺法

GB/T 21709.21-2013　针灸技术操作规范第21部分：毫针基本手法

GB/T 30232-2013　针灸学通用术语

GB/T 40997-2021　经外奇穴名称与定位

3　术语和定义

下列术语和定义适用于本文件。

3.1

醒脑开窍针刺法

通过针刺水沟、内关、三阴交为代表的组方腧穴，并施用特定手法，复苏受抑制、受损伤的脑组织功能，并恢复其传导、联络与支配作用的治疗方法。

3.2

中风

由于脏腑虚衰，情志变动，外因诱发等，致使风痰入络，或气血逆乱，脑络痹阻，或血溢于脑，引发以突然昏仆，或半身不遂，口眼㖞斜，肢体麻木，舌謇难言等为特征的颅脑病。

　　［来源：GB/T 16751.1-1997，8.1.1，有修改］

3.3

雀啄泻法

进针后，施以单向捻转，使肌纤维缠绕针体，再施以像鸟雀啄食般上下运动的行针手法。

注：注意针体与皮肤不可发生位移。

3.4

下极泉

在臂前区，极泉与少海连线上，极泉下1~2寸，避开腋毛，肌肉丰厚处。

注：极泉穴处腋毛浓密，汗腺发达，不易消毒，易发生感染，加之极泉穴外侧为腋动脉且局部组织疏松，易引
发血肿，故醒脑开窍针刺法用下极泉穴替代极泉穴。

3.5

上八邪

在手背，当第2~5掌指关节间上1寸，左右共6穴。

3.6

捻转提插结合泻法

以任脉、督脉为纵轴，以患者体位区分左右，捻转时拇指作用力方向为左侧逆时针、右侧顺时
针，同时施以轻插重提的手法。

4 施术前准备

4.1 针具选择

a）一次性毫针应符合GB 2024-2016规定。

b）根据病情和操作部位选择不同型号的毫针。

c）选择针身光滑、无锈蚀和折痕，针柄牢固，针尖锐利、无倒钩的针具。

4.2 体位选择

选择患者感觉舒适、医者便于操作的体位，应符合GB/T 21709.20-2009规定。

4.3 腧穴定位

参见GB/T 12346-2021经穴名称与定位、GB/T 40997-2021经外奇穴名称与定位。

4.4 消毒

针具器械消毒、接触物品消毒、医者手消毒、针刺部位消毒以及对治疗室、备品的要求，均应
符合GB 15982-2012的规定。

4.5 环境要求

治疗环境应安静，清洁卫生，光线充足，温度适宜。

5 主穴

5.1 治疗原则

醒脑开窍，滋补肝脾肾。

5.2 应用范围

a）主穴Ⅰ：中风后尚未接受醒脑开窍针刺法治疗的患者，宜至少连续应用主穴Ⅰ治疗3次；中
风后意识障碍患者，宜用主穴Ⅰ治疗直至意识清醒。

b）主穴Ⅱ：中风后意识清醒，且出现主动运动的患者，宜用主穴Ⅱ治疗。

c）主穴Ⅰ、主穴Ⅱ交替应用：中风后意识清醒，但主动运动尚未出现的患者，宜交替应用主穴
Ⅰ、主穴Ⅱ进行治疗。

5.3 主穴Ⅰ操作

5.3.1 腧穴组成

内关、水沟、三阴交。

5.3.2 操作步骤与要求

5.3.2.1 医者面向患者，按内关、水沟、三阴交的顺序进行针刺，具体操作如下。

5.3.2.2 内关：单手进针，直刺0.5~1寸，采用捻转提插结合泻法，双侧同时操作，施术1 min，不
留针。

5.3.2.3 水沟：单手进针，向鼻中隔方向斜刺0.3~0.5寸，采用雀啄泻法，以眼球湿润或流泪为度，留针30 min。

5.3.2.4 三阴交：无下肢功能障碍患者，取双侧三阴交，单手进针，直刺1~1.5寸，采用捻转补法，双侧同时操作，施手法1 min，留针30 min；合并下肢功能障碍患者，取患侧三阴交，单手进针，沿胫骨内侧面后缘进针，针体与胫骨内侧面呈45°，刺入0.5~1寸，采用提插补法，以患侧下肢抽动3次为度，不留针。

5.4 主穴Ⅱ操作

5.4.1 腧穴组成

内关、印堂、上星、三阴交。

5.4.2 操作步骤与要求

5.4.2.1 按内关、印堂、上星、三阴交的顺序进行针刺，具体操作如下。

5.4.2.2 内关：操作见5.3.2.2。

5.4.2.3 印堂：取提捏进针法，向鼻尖方向平刺0.3~0.5寸，采用雀啄泻法，施手法1 min，留针30 min。

5.4.2.4 上星：取夹持进针法，向百会方向透刺2.5寸，采用平补平泻手法，施手法1 min，留针30 min。

5.4.2.5 三阴交：操作见5.3.2.4。

6 辅穴

6.1 治疗原则

补益脑髓，疏通经络。

6.2 应用范围

辅穴配合主穴应用于以下情况：

a）辅穴Ⅰ：适用于所有中风患者，尤其适用于椎基底动脉供血不足患者。

b）辅穴Ⅱ：适用于中风合并肢体功能障碍的患者。

6.3 辅穴Ⅰ操作

6.3.1 腧穴组成

风池、完骨、天柱。

6.3.2 操作步骤与要求

6.3.2.1 按风池、完骨、天柱的顺序进行针刺，具体操作如下。

6.3.2.2 风池：单手进针，向对侧眼球方向直刺1~1.5寸，施用小幅度、高频率捻转补法，双侧同时操作，施手法1 min，留针30 min。

6.3.2.3 完骨、天柱：单手进针，直刺1~1.5寸，施用小幅度、高频率捻转补法，双侧同时操作，每穴施手法1 min，留针30 min。

注：小幅度、高频率捻转补法，指捻转幅度小于90°、频率在120~160次/分的行针手法。

6.4 辅穴Ⅱ操作

6.4.1 腧穴组成

下极泉、尺泽、委中。

6.4.2 操作步骤与要求

6.4.2.1 按下极泉、尺泽、委中的顺序进行针刺，具体操作如下。

6.4.2.2 下极泉：使患侧上肢外展90°，充分暴露下极泉，单手进针，直刺1~1.5寸，采用提插泻法，以患侧上肢抽动3次为度，不留针。

6.4.2.3 尺泽：使患侧上肢屈肘120°，单手进针，直刺0.5~0.8寸，采用提插泻法，以患侧前臂、手外旋抽动3次为度，不留针。

6.4.2.4 委中：使患侧下肢抬起呈伸直状态，单手进针，直刺或向外斜刺1~1.5寸，采用提插泻法，以患侧下肢抽动3次为度，不留针。

7 合并症治疗

7.1 吞咽障碍

a）在主穴、辅穴基础上，配合应用点刺咽后壁，针刺风池、完骨、翳风。

b）主穴、辅穴操作同本文件5、6，配穴操作先点刺咽后壁，再按风池、完骨、翳风的顺序进行针刺。

1）咽后壁：嘱患者抬头张口，医者用压舌板将舌体压下，使咽后壁充分暴露，以毫针在咽后壁点刺8~10次。

2）风池、完骨、翳风：单手进针，均向喉结方向直刺2~2.5寸，采用小幅度、高频率捻转补法，双侧同时操作，每穴施手法1 min，留针30 min。

7.2 语言障碍

a）在主穴、辅穴基础上，配合应用针刺金津、玉液，点刺舌面。

b）主穴、辅穴操作同本文件5、6，配穴操作按金津、玉液、舌面的顺序进行点刺。

1）金津、玉液：用舌钳或无菌纱布将患者舌体拉起，以三棱针点刺，出血1~3 ml，术后嘱患者温水漱口。

2）舌面：嘱患者抬头张口，以毫针在舌面散刺8~10次。

7.3 肩手综合征

a）在主穴、辅穴基础上，配合应用肩髃、肩髎、肩贞、肩中俞、肩外俞、阿是穴。

b）主穴、辅穴操作同本文件5、6，配穴操作先针刺腧穴，起针后再进行阿是穴刺络拔罐。

1）肩髃、肩髎、肩贞：均取患侧，单手进针，直刺1~1.5寸，采用提插泻法，每穴施手法1 min，留针30 min。

2）肩中俞、肩外俞：均取患侧，单手进针，斜刺0.5~0.8寸，采用提插泻法，每穴施手法1 min，留针30 min。

3）阿是穴：使患侧上肢被动运动，寻找肩部痛点，三棱针点刺3~5次后拔罐，适量出血3~5 ml，留罐时间不宜超过5 min。

7.4 手指功能障碍

a）在主穴、辅穴基础上，配合应用合谷、上八邪。

b）主穴、辅穴操作同本文件5、6，配穴操作按合谷、上八邪的顺序进行针刺。

1）合谷：取患侧，单手进针，向三间方向斜刺1~1.5寸，采用提插泻法，以患者紧握的手指自然伸展或食指不自主抽动3次为度；另取1支毫针，仍在合谷位置，向第1掌指关节基底部斜刺1~1.5寸，采用提插泻法，以拇指抽动3次为度，留针30 min。

2）上八邪：取患侧，单手进针，向掌指关节基底部斜刺1~1.5寸，采用提插泻法，以手指抽动3次为度，留针30 min。

7.5 足内翻

a）在主穴、辅穴基础上，配合应用丘墟。

b）主穴、辅穴操作同本文件5、6，配穴操作：将患足摆放至功能位，一手固定患足，另一手持针自丘墟向照海方向缓慢透刺，针体从踝关节的骨缝间隙穿过，进针2~2.5寸，在照海部位看到皮肤鼓起但针尖不刺破皮肤，且以患足出现背屈为度，然后将针体退至皮下1寸，留针30 min。

> **注**：此施术过程，动作应轻柔缓慢。须固定患者膝关节，避免患侧下肢、足踝出现屈曲反射将针体夹弯，甚至出现折针或断针。

8 注意事项

a）饥饿、饱食、醉酒、大怒、大惊、过度疲劳、精神紧张者，不宜立即进行针刺；体质虚弱、气血亏损者，其针感不宜过重，应尽量采取卧位行针。

b）施术过程中，术者手指需要触及针体时，应用消毒棉球作间隔物，术者手指不宜直接接触针体。

c）胸背部腧穴，不宜深刺，避免气胸。

d）刺血施术时，医者应戴医用手套避免接触患者血液。

e）对于易出血部位，出针后宜用干棉球按压一定时间，不宜擦揉。

9 禁忌

a）皮肤有感染、溃疡、瘢痕或肿瘤的部位，禁用针刺。

b）有凝血缺陷的患者，禁用针刺。

c）脑出血活动期、恶性高血压的患者，禁用水沟穴。

d）妊娠期中风患者，禁用合谷、三阴交等对胎孕反应敏感的腧穴。

e）不能配合施术的患者，禁用针刺。

附录 A

（资料性）

醒脑开窍针刺法的含义

"醒"，本义指睡眠状态的结束，与"睡"相对，《灵枢》言"明于阴阳，如惑之解，如醉之醒"。引申义：一是"清醒"，指思维意识的正常状态；二是"苏醒"，指思维意识由昏愦、朦胧逐渐转为清醒状态；三是"复苏"，指曾经一度受抑、受损、受挫的功能活动，重新得以恢复。醒脑开窍法的"醒"字，主要指"复苏"之义。

"开"与"醒"意思相近，有启闭、开发之义。

"神"，生命活动的总称。中医的"神"有狭义和广义之分，狭义之"神"，仅指思维、意识、精神状态、认知能力等；广义之"神"，在人体生命科学中即指人体生命的一切功能活动的能力，以及通过各种功能活动而产生的有形物质的外部征象。人能视物辨味、站立行走、感受自然、认知社会和五脏六腑功能正常运转均为"神"所主，正如《素问·灵兰秘典》所云："主明则下安。主不明则十二官危，脉道闭塞，形乃大伤。"明代李时珍云："脑为元神之府。"《元气论》云："脑实则神全，神全则气全，气全则形全，形全则百关调于内，邪消于外。"可见，神藏于脑，脑为"神明之体"。由于脑与神的密切关系，所以"醒脑"亦可称为"醒神"。

"窍"，《黄帝内经》中窍有二义：其一，指"孔窍"，如口鼻、前后阴等；其二，指"通路""关口"之义，用以说明其传导、支配作用畅通与否，多为后世医论中的"心窍""脑窍""神窍"等。醒脑开窍法的"窍"，是指脑、神的通路，即"脑窍""神窍"。

综上，醒脑开窍是指复苏人体脑窍及其连属组织的受抑制、受损伤的功能，并开发、恢复其传导、联络和支配作用的治疗方法。

基于对中风病因病机的充分认识和广义之神的深刻理解，石学敏院士提出了中风的根本病机是"窍闭神匿，神不导气"，确立了"醒脑开窍、滋补肝脾肾、补益脑髓、疏通经络"的治则，醒神调神为"使"，开窍启闭为"用"，从脑论治中风，创立了以取阴经及督脉经穴为主的"醒脑开窍"针刺法理论和技术体系。

参 考 文 献

［1］ 石学敏.脑卒中与醒脑开窍（第2版）［M］.北京：科学出版社，2015.

［2］ 石学敏.国医大师石学敏学术与临床集锦［M］.北京：中国医药科技出版社，2018.

［3］ 胡国强，石学敏."醒脑开窍法"治疗中风手法量学的基础研究［J］.中国针灸，1992；12（2）：33.

［4］ 石学敏.中风病与醒脑开窍针刺法［M］.天津：天津科学技术出版社，1998：198.

Foreword

Please note that parts of this document may involve patent rights. The issuing organization for this document shall not be held responsible for identifying any or all such patent rights.

Main drafting unit: First Affiliated Hospital of Tianjin University of Traditional Chinese Medicine, National Clinical Research Center for Traditional Chinese Acupuncture and Moxibustion.

Other involved drafting units (In no particular order): Chongqing Traditional Chinese Medicine Hospital, Ningxia Hui Autonomous Region Traditional Chinese Medicine Hospital and Academy of Traditional Chinese Medicine, Shenzhen Bao'an Hospital of Traditional Chinese Medicine, Arizona Acupuncture Institute and Chinese Herbal Medicine (U.S.A.), Maidstone Chinese Medical Centre (United Kingdom), Chinese Medicine Clinic in Munich (Germany), National Cancer Institute (Malaysia).

Main Drafter: Shi Xuemin.

Other involved drafters and reviewers (In pinyin alphabetical order by surname):

China: Bian Jinling, Chang Yinghui, Dai Xiaoyu, Du Yuzheng, Guo Yang, Li Li, Liu Jian, Shi Huiyan, Wang Can, Wang Zhuxing, Xiao Lingyong, Yu Lan, Zhang Chao, Zhao Qi.

U.S.A: Liu Jing.

Britain: Zhao Junhong.

Germany: Florian von Damnitz.

Malaysia: Zhong Shangye.

The drafting procedure for this document adheres to the standards contained within *Managing Principles for Organizational Standards of the World Federation of Chinese Medicine Societies*, and SCM 0001-2009 *Working Regulations for Standards Formulation and Publication*, issued by the World Federation of Chinese Medicine Societies (WFCMS).

Introduction

This document serves to standardize the clinical Xingnao Kaiqiao acupuncture manipulations (invigorate the brain and open the orifices). As a guide to assist relevant practitioners in appropriately applying the techniques, it ensures proper utilization of the Xingnao Kaiqiao techniques within domains of clinical application, education, and research. The standards contained in this document also serves to ensure the safety and efficacy of Xingnao Kaiqiao techniques, in order to better facilitate their international propagation and application.

Needling technique is the key to producing good clinical results through acupuncture treatment, with the degree of stimulation being the primary factor in affecting clinical efficacy. Physicians throughout history have conducted simple quantitative analyses of needling technique, mostly relying on subjective experience and lacking in mature and unified objective quantitative standards. In 1976, Academician Shi Xuemin first proposed the concept of studying needling techniques in a quantitative manner. This was the first time that the four major elements of needling techniques were scientifically defined, including direction and magnitude of needling acting force, time of treatment, and time between treatments. These definitions have rendered needling techniques more standardized, repeatable, and operable.

There are a number of parameters involved when discussing needling technique, including stimulation, insertion (direction, angle, depth), timing (time of intervention, length of manipulation, needle retention, frequency, treatment course, etc.), and manipulation (manual technique, range, frequency, etc.). Early clinical studies have showed that when comparing the utilization of standardized quantitative needling techniques to those of non-standardized quantitative needling techniques, stroke patients who received standardized techniques exhibited greater improvement in terms of electroencephalogram, cerebral blood flow, microcirculation, blood rheology and other indicators, thus leading to better restoration of motor, sensory, and language functions. Recent functional imaging studies have noted that needling technique is the key influential factor in affecting brain functional imaging changes. Fundamental research has also shown that length of manipulation and frequency of needle rotation are important factors influencing treatment efficacy. Each parameter also has its own specific biological pathway(s) for regulation.

Therefore, scientifically established standards of quantitative needling techniques are necessary conditions in ensuring maximal treatment efficacy. The development of studies in quantitative needle techniques is a necessary path to standardization of acupuncture.

International Standardized Manipulations of Chinese Medicine Xingnao Kaiqiao Acupuncture for Stroke

1 Scope

This document specifies the terms and definitions, treatment principles, scope of application, acupoint combinations, operational steps and requirements, precautions and contraindications of Xingnao Kaiqiao acupuncture for stroke.

This document is applicable to the clinical technical operation of Xingnao Kaiqiao acupuncture for stroke.

2 Normative references

The contents of the following documents constitute essential provisions of this document through normative references in-text. For dated references, only the version corresponding to the specified date applies to this document. For undated references, the latest version (including all amendments) applies to this document.

GB 2024-2016　Acupuncture Needles

GB/T 12346-2021　Nomenclature and location of meridian points

GB 15982-2012　Hygienic standard for disinfection in hospitals

GB/T 16751.1-1997　Clinic terminology of traditional Chinese medical diagnosis and treatment. Part 1: Disease

GB/T 21709.4-2008　Standardized manipulations of acupuncture and moxibustion. Part 4: Three-edged needle

GB/T 21709.20-2009　Standardized manipulations of acupuncture and moxibustion. Part 20: Basic techniques of filiform needle

GB/T 21709.21-2013　Standardized manipulations of acupuncture and moxibustion. Part 21: Filiform needle manipulation by basic applying technique

GB/T 30232-2013　General nomenclature of science of acupuncture and moxibustion

GB/T 40997-2021　Nomenclature and location of extra points in common use

3 Terms and definitions

The following terms and definitions apply to this document.

3.1

Xingnao Kaiqiao acupuncture

Treatment method consisting of specific manipulations at acupoint combination prescriptions constituted by Shuigou (GV26), Neiguan (PC6) and Sanyinjiao (SP6), to revive the functions of inhibited and damaged brain tissue, and to restore its conduction, communication and control functions.

3.2

Stroke

A craniocerebral disease characterized by symptoms including sudden loss of consciousness, hemiplegia, facial or ocular deviation, numbness in the body or extremities, disarthria and aphasia. Risk factors include viscera deficiency, emotional disturbances, or external factors, which can cause wind phlegm invasion of collaterals, qi and blood disorder, brain collateral obstruction, or overflow of blood into the brain.

[Source: GB/T 16751.1-1997, 8.1.1 modified]

3.3

Sparrow-pecking (que zhuo) reduction technique

Needling technique involving application of post-insertion uni-directional twisting so that muscle fibers wrap around the body of the needle, followed by lifting-thrusting oscillations which mimic the pecking of a sparrow.

Note: Care should be taken not to displace the needle body and the skin.

3.4

Lower Jiquan (lower HT1)

This acupoint is located in the brachial region, on the line between Jiquan (HT1) and Shaohai (HT3), 1-2 cun below Jiquan (HT1). Locate this acupoint in the dense muscular area while avoiding the axillary hair.

Note: The location of Jiquan (HT1) is characterized by dense axillary hair and developed sweat glands, which can be difficult to disinfect. Acupuncture on Jiguan (HT1) may easily cause infection. Hematoma occurrences are also increased by having the axillary artery being just lateral to Jiquan (HT1), as well as Jiquan (HT1) having slack local tissue, so lower Jiquan (lower HT1) is often used as a substitute to Jiquan (HT1).

3.5

Upper Baxie (upper EX-UE9)

Located on the dorsum of the hand, 1 cun proximal to the spaces between the second to fifth metacarpophalangeal joints. There are 6 points in total when counting both hands.

3.6

Twirling and lifting-thrusting combined reduction technique

A manipulation which takes Du and Ren channels as vertical axes, and divides the patient body into left and right based on patient body position. The technique involves performing left counterclockwise and right clockwise rotations based on the direction of thumb movement, combined with light thrusting and vigorous lifting.

4 Preparations before treatment

4.1 Needle selection

a) Disposable filiform needles shall comply with the provisions of GB 2024-2016.

b) Appropriate filiform needles shall be selected according to the patient condition and site of operation.

c) Choose needles with smooth bodies, no rust and bends, with firm handles, sharp tips, and lack of barbs.

4.2 Posture selection

Choose a position that is comfortable for the patient, convenient for the performing doctor, and which complies with the provisions of GB/T 21709.20-2009.

4.3 Acupoint positioning

Refer to GB/T 12346-2021 and GB/T 40997-2021.

4.4 Disinfection

Disinfection should be performed on needles and equipment, contact items, doctors' hands, acupuncture sites, and requirements for treatment rooms and spare supplies; procedures should all meet the requirements of GB 15982-2012.

4.5 Treatment area requirements

The treatment area should be quiet, clean and hygienic, with sufficient light and suitable temperature.

5 Primary acupoints

5.1 Treatment principles

Xingnao kaiqiao (Invigorate the brain and open the orifices), and nourish liver, spleen, and kidney.

5.2 Scope of application

a) Primary acupoints–Set Ⅰ : Indicated for stroke patients who have not yet received Xingnao kaiqiao acupuncture treatment. Such patients should be treated at least 3 times continuously with Set Ⅰ . Stroke patients with impaired consciousness should be treated with Set I until consciousness returns.

b) Primary acupoints–Set Ⅱ : Indicated for conscious stroke patients who exhibit voluntary movement.

c) Alternation of Set Ⅰ and Set Ⅱ : Indicated for conscious stroke patients who have not yet exhibited voluntary movement.

5.3 Technique for primary acupoints-Set Ⅰ

5.3.1 Acupoint composition

Neiguan (PC6), Shuigou (GV26), Sanyinjiao (SP6).

5.3.2 Operational procedures and requirements

5.3.2.1 While facing the patient, acupuncture should be performed on Neiguan (PC6), Shuigou (GV26), and Sanyinjiao (SP6) in order. Specific operational procedure is as follows.

5.3.2.2 Neiguan (PC6): Insertion should be performed with one hand, directed 0.5-1 cun perpendicularly. Twirling and lifting-thrusting reduction technique should be utilized bilaterally at the same time for 1 minute, without retaining needles.

5.3.2.3 Shuigou (GV26): Insertion should be performed with one hand, directed obliquely towards the nasal septum 0.3-0.5 cun. Sparrow-pecking reduction technique should be utilized until eyeballs are moist or tearful. Retain needles for 30 minutes.

5.3.2.4 Sanyinjiao (SP6): For patients without lower extremity dysfunction, insertion should be performed bilaterally, each with one hand, directed perpendicularly 1-1.5 cun; twirling reinforcing technique should be utilized bilaterally at the same time for 1 minute; retain needles for 30 minutes. For patients with lower extremity dysfunction, perform insertion on the affected side with one hand; the needle should be inserted along the medial-posterior side of the tibia, with the needle being 45° to the medial-posterior tibia, at a depth of 0.5-1 cun; lifting-thrusting reinforcing technique should be utilized, until the affected lower extremity twitches 3 times, without retaining needles.

5.4 Technique for primary acupoints-Set Ⅱ

5.4.1 Acupoint composition

Neiguan (PC6), Yintang (GV24⁺), Shangxing (GV23), Sanyinjiao (SP6).

5.4.2 Operational procedures and requirements

5.4.2.1 Acupuncture should be performed on Neiguan (PC6), Yintang (GV24⁺), Shangxing (GV23), Sanyinjiao (SP6) in order. Specific operational procedure is as follows.

5.4.2.2 Neiguan (PC6): Refer to 5.3.2.2 for technique.

5.4.2.3 Yintang (GV24⁺): Lift and pinch the treatment area prior to insertion, and insert 0.3-0.5 cun towards the tip of the nose. Sparrow-pecking reduction technique should be utilized for 1 minute. Retain needle for 30 minutes.

5.4.2.4 Shangxing (GV23): Utilize the clamp-hold insertion method, insert 2.5 cun towards Baihui (GV20). Utilize neutral reinforcing-reducing technique for 1 minute and retain needle for 30 minutes.

5.4.2.5 Sanyinjiao (SP6): Refer to 5.3.2.4 for technique.

6 Auxiliary acupoints

6.1 Treatment principles

Tonify and nourish brain marrow, dredge and clear meridians.

6.2 Scope of application

The auxiliary acupoints are to be combined with primary acupoints in the following situations.

a) Auxiliary acupoints–Set Ⅰ: Indicated for all types of stroke patients, especially for vertebrobasilar artery insufficiency patients.

b) Auxiliary acupoints–Set Ⅱ: Indicated for stroke patients with limb dysfunction.

6.3 Technique for auxiliary acupoints-Set Ⅰ

6.3.1 Acupoint composition

Fengchi (GB20), Wangu (GB12), Tianzhu (BL10).

6.3.2 Operational procedures and requirements

6.3.2.1 Acupuncture should be performed on Fengchi (GB20), Wangu (GB12), Tianzhu (BL10) in order. Specific operational procedure is as follows.

6.3.2.2 Fengchi (GB20): Perpendicular insertion with one hand towards the contralateral eyeball, 1-1.5 cun. Utilize low amplitude, high frequency twirling reinforcing manipulations bilaterally at the same time for 1 minute, and retain needles for 30 minutes.

6.3.2.3 Wangu (GB12), Tianzhu (BL10): Perpendicular insertion with one hand at a depth of 1-1.5 cun. Utilize low amplitude, high frequency twirling reinforcing manipulations bilaterally at the same time for 1 minute at each point, and retain needles for 30 minutes.

> **Note:** Parameters of low amplitude, high frequency twirling reinforcing manipulations include finger rotations of less than 90°, and frequencies of between 120-160 times per minute.

6.4 Technique for auxiliary acupoints-Set Ⅱ

6.4.1 Acupoint composition

Lower Jiquan (lower HT1), Chize (LU5), Weizhong (BL40).

6.4.2 Operational procedures and requirements

6.4.2.1 Acupuncture should be performed on Lower Jiquan (lower HT1), Chize (LU5), Weizhong

(BL40) in order. Specific operational procedure is as follows:

6.4.2.2 Lower Jiquan (lower HT1):Abduct the affected upper limb to 90° to fully expose Lower Jiquan (lower HT1). Insert with one hand in a perpendicular direction to a depth of 1-1.5 cun, apply lifting-thrusting reduction manipulations, until the affected upper limb twitches 3 times. Do not retain needles.

6.4.2.3 Chize (LU5): Flex the affected elbow to 120°. Insert with one hand in a perpendicular direction to a depth of 0.5-0.8 cun, applying lifting-thrusting reduction manipulations, until the affected forearm and hand rotates externally 3 times. Do not retain needles.

6.4.2.4 Weizhong (BL40): Lift and fully extend the affected lower limb. Insertwith one hand in a perpendicular or obliquely outwards to a depth of 1-1.5 cun, apply lifting-thrusting reduction manipulations, until the affected lower limb twitches 3 times. Do not retain needles.

7 Treatment for complications

7.1 Dysphagia

a) On the basis of the primary and auxiliary acupoints, incorporate pricking on the posterior pharyngeal wall, along with needling of Fengchi (GB20), Wangu (GB12) and Yifeng (TE17).

b) Operation of primary and auxiliary acupoints should follow items 5 and 6 of this document. Treatment technique for dysphagia should first involve pricking of the posterior pharyngeal wall, followed by needling at Fengchi (GB20), Wangu (GB12), and Yifeng (SJ17) in order. Specific operational procedure is as follows.

1) Posterior pharyngeal wall: Ask the patient to raise the head and open the mouth. Use a tongue depressor to hold down the tongue and expose the posterior pharyngeal wall. Prick the posterior pharyngeal wall 8-10 times with a filiform needle.

2) Fengchi (GB20), Wangu (GB12) and Yifeng (SJ17): Insert with one hand in a perpendicular direction towards the laryngeal prominence, to a depth of 2-2.5 cun. Apply lower amplitude, high frequency twirling reinforcing technique, bilaterally at the same time, for 1 minute at each acupoint. Retain needles for 30 minutes.

7.2 Aphasia

a) On the basis of the primary and auxiliary acupoints, incorporate needling at Jinjin (EX-HN12), Yuye (EX-HN13), as well as pricking of the lingual surface.

b) Operation of primary and auxiliary acupoints should follow items 5 and 6 of this document. Treatment technique for aphasia should involve needling at Jinjin (EX-HN12), Yuye (EX-HN13), and lingual surface in order. Specific operational procedure is as follows.

1) Jinjin (EX-HN12), Yuye (EX-HN13): Hold and raise the patient's tongue with tongue forceps or sterile gauze, then prick and bleed with a three-edged needle until 1-3ml of blood is extracted. Ask patient to rinse mouth with warm water after the procedure.

2) Lingual surface: Ask patient to raise the head and open the mouth, and perform 8-10 scattered pricks on the lingual surface with a filiform needle.

7.3 Shoulder-hand syndrome

7.3.1 Acupoint composition

Jianyu (LI15), Jianliao (TE14), Jianzhen (SI9), Jianzhongshu (SI15), Jianwaishu (SI14), Ashi points

7.3.2 Operational procedures and requirements

a) On the basis of the primary and auxiliary acupoints, incorporate the use of Jianyu (LI15), Jianliao (TE14), Jianzhen (SI9), Jianzhongshu (SI15), Jianwaishu (SI14), and Ashi points.

b) Operation of primary and auxiliary acupoints should follow items 5 and 6 of this document. Treatment for shoulder-hand syndrome should involve needling at the 5 acupoints, followed by collateral pricking and cupping at the Ashi points:

1) Jianyu (LI15), Jianliao (TE14), Jianzhen (SI9): On the affected side, insert with one hand in a perpendicular direction at a depth of 1-1.5 cun. Apply lifting-thrusting reduction manipulation, 1 minute per acupoint. Retain needles for 30 minutes.

2) Jianzhongshu (SI15), Jianwaishu (SI14): On the affected side, insert with one hand in an oblique direction at a depth of 0.5-0.8 cun. Apply lifting-thrusting reduction manipulation, 1 minute per acupoint. Retain needles for 30 minutes.

3) Ashi points: Passively move the affected upper limb and look for Ashi points in the shoulder. Prick 3-5 times with a three-edged needle, followed by cupping until 3-5ml of blood is extracted. Do not retain cups for more than 5 minutes.

7.4 Finger function impairment

7.4.1 Acupoint composition

Hegu (LI4), Upper Baxie (Upper EX-UE9).

7.4.2 Operational procedures and requirements

a) On the basis of the primary and auxiliary acupoints, incorporate the use of Hegu (LI4) and Upper Baxie (Upper EX-UE9).

b) Operation of primary and auxiliary acupoints should follow items 5 and 6 of this document. Treatment technique for finger function impairment should involve needling at Hegu (LI4) and Upper Baxie (Upper EX-UE9)in order. Specific operational procedure is as follows.

1) Hegu (LI4): On the affected side, insert with one hand in an oblique direction towards Sanjian (LI3), at a depth of 1-1.5 cun. Apply lifting-thrusting reduction manipulation, until tightly flexed fingers extend naturally or until index finger twitches 3 times. Next, insert another needle at Hegu (LI4) obliquely towards the base of the first metacarpal joint, at a depth of 1-1.5 cun. Apply lifting-thrusting reduction manipulations until thumb twitches 3 times. Retain needles for 30 minutes.

2) Upper Baxie (Upper EX-UE9): On the affected side, insert with one hand in an oblique direction towards the base of the metacarpal joint, at a depth of 1-1.5 cun. Apply lifting-thrusting manipulations until the fingers twitch 3 times. Retain needles for 30 minutes.

7.5 Strephenopodia

7.5.1 Acupoint composition

Qiuxu (GB40).

7.5.2 Operational procedures and requirements

a) On the basis of the primary and auxiliary acupoints, incorporate the use of Qiuxu (GB40).

b) Operation of primary and auxiliary acupoints should follow items 5 and 6 of this document. Treatment technique for strephenopodia involves placing the affected foot in a normal physiological position and fixing it with one hand. Insert at Qiuxu (GB40) with the other hand slowly towards in the direction of Zhaohai (KI6), so that the needle passes between the bones of the ankle joint, at a depth of

2-2.5 cun. At Zhaohai (KI6) the skin should appear raised, but the needle should not puncture the skin, and the affected foot should exhibit dorsiflexion. Next, draw out the needle until it is just 1 cun under the skin, and retain needles for 30 minutes.

> **Note:** During this procedure, the movements should be gentle, soft, and slow. The patient's knee needs to be stabilized, as to avoid flexion of the affected lower limbs or ankle which will bend the needle body, possibly leading to a bent or broken needle.

8 Precautions

a) Patients who are hungry, full, intoxicated, furious, frightened, overly fatigued, or mentally nervous should not be treated immediately. Patients with weak constitutions or deficiencies of qi and blood should not be subjected to strong deqi sensations, and should be in supine lying position during the treatment.

b) If the practitioner needs to touch the needle body during the procedure, a sterile cotton ball should be used as a buffer, and the practitioners' fingers shall not directly touch the needle body.

c) Acupoints on the chest and back should not be needled too deeply in order to avoid pneumothorax.

d) During the pricking procedure, the practitioners should wear medical gloves to avoid contact with patients' blood.

e) For areas prone to bleeding, it is advisable to apply pressure to the point with a dry cotton ball for a set amount of time after needle removal, and not to rub the area.

9 Contraindications

a) Acupuncture is contraindicated on skin areas with infection, ulcers, scars or tumors.

b) Acupuncture is contraindicated for patients with coagulation problems.

c) Shuigou (GV26) is contraindicated in patients with active cerebral hemorrhage and malignant hypertension.

d) Acupoints which pregnantwomen are sensitive to, including Hegu (LI4) and Sanyinjiao (SP6), etc., are contraindicated for pregnant stroke patients.

e) Acupuncture is contraindicated for patients who cannot cooperate with the procedures.

Annex A
(Informative)
Explanation of Xingnao Kaiqiao Acupuncture

The original meaning of "Xing" refers to state that the spleeping state just ends. *The Lingshu* (*Spiritual Pivot*) states that "Understanding yin and yang is akin to finding resolution in confusion, like sobering from a drunken stupor". There are several extended meanings of the character "Xing". Firstly it refers to the normal state of consciousness, "Qing xing". The second meaning is "to awaken", or "Su xing", which refers to the gradual change of consciousness from being dim and hazy to being in a sober state. The third meaning is "Fu su", which refers to the resuscitation of functions and activities which were once suppressed or damaged. The character "Xing" from "Xingnao Kaiqiao" primarily refers to the third meaning.

"Kai" shares a similar meaning to "Xing", and refers to the opening of obstruction.

"Shen" is the general term for life activities. The term "Shen" in traditional Chinese medicine has a narrow and broad definition. The narrow definition of "Shen" refers to thought processes, consciousness, mental states, cognitive function, etc., while the broad definition of "Shen" refers to all functional and movement abilities of human life within the realm of human life sciences, as well as external signs of tangible matter produced through various functions and activities. "Shen" governs the abilities of humans to see, to differentiate taste and smells, to stand and to walk, to feel and sense the natural world, in addition to the regular functioning of the five zang and six fu organs. As stated in *the Suwen – Linglan Midian Lun* (*Spiritual Pivot – Discussion of the Secret Canons from the Spiritual Terrace and Orchid Chamber*), "An enlightened ruler ensures peaceful subjects; an unenlightened ruler endangers the twelve officials, blocks the meridian pathways, and seriously damages the physical body". Li Shizhen of the Ming dynasty had stated "The brain is the fu organ of the congenital spirit". The *Yuan Qi Lun* (*Discussion of Congenital Qi*) states that "When the brain becomes full, then the Shen is complete; if the Shen is complete then qi is complete; if the qi is complete then the form is complete; if the form is complete then all hundred gates in the interior are regulated, and the pathogenic factors are expelled outwardly". These descriptions denote that Shen is retained in the brain, and the brain is "the manifestation of the enlightened spirit". Due to this close relationship between the brain and the Shen, "Xingnao" (Resuscitation of the brain) is also known as "Xing Shen" (Resuscitation of the spirit).

The character "Qiao" has two meanings in the *Huangdi Neijing* (*Yellow Emperor's Inner Classic*): the first refers to "hole or orifice", such as the mouth, nose, anterior and posterior genitals, etc.; the second refers to "pathway" or "pass", etc., in relation to the smoothness of conductive or control functions in various pathways. "Qiao" is used in "Xingnao Kaiqiao" in reference to the pathways of the brain and Shen, specifically "nao qiao" (pathway of the brain) and "Shen qiao" (pathway of Shen).

In conclusion, "Xingnao kaiqiao" is a treatment method involved in the resuscitation of the human brain pathway along with its inhibited and damaged functions, through opening and restoration of conductive, communicative, and control functions.

Based on a comprehensive grasp of the etiology and pathogenesis of stroke, as well as a deep understanding of the broad definition of "Shen", Academician Shi Xuemin proposed that the fundamental pathogenesis of stroke is "Closing of the pathways and inhibition of Shen, such that Shen does not guide the qi". His proposed pathogenesis gave rise to the treatment principles "Xingnao kaiqiao; tonify the liver, spleen and kidney; nourish the brain marrow; dredge the channels and collaterals". The resuscitation and regulation of Shen are the "envoys", while the opening of orifice pathways is the "application". His approach treats stroke from the perspective of the brain, and establishes "Xingnao Kaiqiao" acupuncture theories and techniques which primarily choose the acupoints on Yin meridians and Du meridian.

References

［1］ Shi Xuemin, Stroke and Xingnao Kaiqiao (2nd edition)[M]. Beijing: Science Press. 2015.

［2］ Shi Xuemin, Collection of Academic and Clinical Discussion of Academic National Grandmaster Shi Xuemin[M]. Beijing: China Medical Science and Technology Publishing House, 2018.

［3］ Hu Guoqiang, Shi Xuemin. "Fundamental Research on the Quantification of Manipulating Techniques of Resuscitating Method for Restoration of Consciousness in the Treatment of Apoplexy" [J]. China Acupuncture and Moxibustion, 1992; 12(2):33.

［4］ Shi Xuemin. Apoplexy and Acupuncture for Refreshing the Brain and Resuscitation[M]. Tianjin: Tianjin Science and Technology Press, 1998:198.